Quick Fit: 21 Days to a Leaner You
Here's a streamlined Table of Contents for your diet eBook, "Quick Fit: 21 Days to a Leaner You," with five chapters to fit the content of a concise three-week program:

Table of Contents

1. **Introduction**
   - Welcome to "Quick Fit: 21 Days to a Leaner You"
   - How to Use This Book
   - What to Expect in the Next 21 Days

2. **Week 1: Building the Foundation**
   - Setting Your Goals and Understanding Nutrition
   - Kickstarting Your Fitness Journey
   - Week 1 Meal Plans and Recipes

This format ensures that each week is covered in detail, providing a step-by-step guide that corresponds to the 21-day structure of the diet program, leading up to a final chapter that helps readers transition to a sustainable lifestyle beyond the duration of the eBook.

Chapter 1: Day 1-7: Laying the Foundations

Welcome to the first week of your journey towards a leaner you! This initial phase is all about establishing a solid foundation for the rest of your 21-day transformation. We'll focus on setting realistic goals, understanding basic nutrition, and easing into an exercise routine that doesn't require hours at the gym.

Setting Your Goals

Start by defining clear, achievable goals. Are you aiming to lose weight, tone up, or both? How much weight do you want to lose this week? Make your goals specific, measurable, achievable, relevant, and time-bound (SMART). For instance, a goal might be, "I want to lose 1 pound by the end of this week by reducing my daily calorie intake and exercising for 30 minutes each day."

Understanding Nutrition

Nutrition is the cornerstone of any effective weight loss program. Focus on consuming a balanced diet rich in vegetables, fruits, lean proteins, and whole grains. Understanding macronutrients—carbohydrates, proteins, and fats—is crucial:

- **Carbohydrates** provide your body with energy. Opt for complex carbs found in whole grains and vegetables over simple carbs like sugar.

- **Proteins** are essential for muscle repair and growth. Include a good protein source in every meal, choosing from lean meats, fish, eggs, or plant-based options like beans and lentils.
- **Fats** are vital for hormonal function and cell health. Choose healthy fats from sources like avocados, nuts, seeds, and olive oil.

This week, try to track your meals either by writing them down or using a food tracking app. This will help you become more aware of what and how much you are eating.

Starting Exercise

In the first week, your exercise routine should be about building the habit of regular physical activity. Aim for at least 150 minutes of moderate-intensity

aerobic activity throughout the week, which you can break down into 30-minute sessions over five days. Here are some activities you might consider:
- Brisk walking or light jogging
- Cycling at a moderate pace
- Swimming gentle laps
- A dance class or online workout video
Include two days of strength training using your body weight or light weights. Exercises like squats, lunges, push-ups, and planks are great starters.
Hydration and Sleep
Drinking enough water is essential, especially as you start exercising more. Aim for at least 8-10 glasses a day. Proper hydration aids in digestion, keeps your energy levels

up, and helps curb unnecessary snacking.

Sleep also plays a critical role in weight loss. It affects your hormones and can impact your hunger and appetite. Try to get between 7-9 hours of quality sleep per night. Establish a calming bedtime routine and try to go to bed and wake up at the same time each day.

Conclusion

The first week is about setting the stage for success. By focusing on smart goal setting, nutritional basics, simple exercises, adequate hydration, and sleep, you're paving the way towards a sustainable transformation. Remember, the changes you make this week will build the foundation for the habits you'll develop over the next two weeks. Keep pushing forward, stay committed, and prepare to see results!

Chapter 2: Day 8-14: Building Momentum

Congratulations on completing your first week! By now, you should be feeling more comfortable with your new routine. This week, we'll build on the foundation you've set and introduce more dynamic exercises, delve deeper into nutrition with meal prepping, and share tips on maintaining hydration.

Enhancing Your Exercise Routine

Now that your body is accustomed to regular physical activity, let's increase the intensity slightly to maximize fat burning and muscle building. You'll continue with the aerobic activities introduced last

week but add some variations and increase the duration slightly if possible. Here's what your exercise plan might look like:
- **Interval Training**: Incorporate short bursts of high-intensity exercise followed by periods of lower intensity or rest. For example, during a 30-minute jog, alternate between jogging for 2 minutes and sprinting for 30 seconds.
- **Strength Training Enhancements**: Add more resistance to your workouts by including weights or resistance bands. Focus on exercises that target multiple muscle groups, such as deadlifts, overhead presses, and pull-ups.
Aim to include at least three days of strength training, alternating with aerobic days to allow your muscles

time to recover. This will not only enhance your muscle tone but also increase your metabolic rate, which helps burn more calories, even at rest.

Advanced Nutrition and Meal Prepping

Nutrition continues to play a crucial role as you intensify your workouts. This week, focus on preparing meals in advance to save time and ensure you always have healthy options on hand. Here's how to get started with meal prepping:

- **Plan Your Meals**: Write down a meal plan for the week. Include all meals and snacks, and make sure each one is balanced with a good mix of carbohydrates, protein, and fats.

- **Batch Cooking**: Select one or two days a week to cook in bulk.

Prepare dishes like grilled chicken, roasted vegetables, and whole grains in large quantities.
- **Smart Storage**: Divide the cooked food into portion-controlled containers. Store them in the refrigerator or freezer based on when you plan to eat them.
This structured approach to eating will help you avoid the temptation of unhealthy snacks and fast food, making it easier to stick to your diet.
Hydration and Its Benefits
As your exercise intensity increases, so does your need for hydration. Water helps transport nutrients in your blood, regulate body temperature, and digest food. It's also crucial for optimal performance during workouts.

- **Set a Water Intake Goal**: Aim for about 2-3 liters of water per day, more if you're sweating heavily during workouts.
- **Monitor Your Hydration**: Pay attention to the color of your urine. It should be light yellow. Dark urine can be a sign of dehydration.

Staying Motivated

Keeping your motivation high is essential as you progress. Here are a few strategies to help keep you driven:

- **Track Your Progress**: Regularly note changes in your weight, body measurements, and how your clothes fit. Also, observe improvements in your physical and mental health.
- **Reward Yourself**: Set small weekly goals and reward yourself for achieving them with non-food

items, like a new workout outfit or a massage.

Conclusion

This week is about taking everything up a notch. By intensifying your workouts, perfecting your meal prepping, and ensuring you stay well-hydrated, you're setting yourself up for even greater success in the final stretch. Remember, consistency is key, and every small effort contributes to major changes. Keep pushing fo Rward!

Chapter 3: Day 15-21: The Home Stretch

You've made it to the final week! Now it's time to push through to the finish line with enhanced strategies and a focus on integrating these changes into your lifestyle.

Maximizing Exercise Impact

Increase the intensity of your workouts this week. Include circuit training, which combines several exercises performed in succession with minimal rest. This will boost your endurance and maximize calorie burn.

Fine-Tuning Nutrition

Focus on fine-tuning your diet. Reduce your intake of processed foods and increase whole foods like fruits, vegetables, and lean proteins, which will help you feel more energized and less bloated.

Mindfulness and Stress Management

Introduce mindfulness practices such as meditation or yoga to manage stress, which can significantly affect weight loss. Taking time to relax and

decompress can prevent overeating caused by stress.
Preparing for Beyond Day 21
Start planning how to maintain these healthy habits beyond the 21 days. Consider how you can incorporate these routines into your daily life to continue seeing results and improving your health.
Finish strong, and remember that this is just the beginning of a healthier, more active lifestyle!
Chapter 4: Maintaining Your Gains
Congratulations on nearing the end of your 21-day journey! This chapter focuses on how to sustain the incredible progress you've made and integrate these healthier habits into your everyday life.
Creating Long-Term Goals

Transition from short-term challenges to long-term goals. Set new objectives for the next three, six, and twelve months. Whether it's improving your personal best in a fitness category, losing additional weight, or simply maintaining your current fitness level, having clear goals will keep you motivated.

Lifestyle Integration

Make exercise and healthy eating a natural part of your daily routine. Schedule workouts as you would any important appointment, and continue planning your meals in advance. This consistency is key to long-term success.

Building a Support Network

Surround yourself with supportive people who encourage your healthy lifestyle. Consider joining fitness groups or online communities where members share similar goals.

Continual Learning and Adaptation

Stay informed about nutrition and fitness. The world of health and wellness is always evolving, so keep learning new techniques and dietary insights to keep your regimen fresh and effective.

By embracing these strategies, you can maintain your gains and enjoy a healthy, vibrant lifestyle indefinitely.

Chapter 5: Recipes and Resources

As you wrap up your 21-day journey, this chapter will provide you with delicious, nutritious recipes and additional resources to keep you motivated and on track.

Healthy Recipes for Continued Success

1. **Morning Boost Smoothie**:
   - 1 cup spinach
   - 1/2 banana
   - 1/2 cup mixed berries
   - 1 tablespoon chia seeds
   - 1 cup almond milk
   Blend all ingredients until smooth for a quick, nutrient-packed breakfast.

2. **Quinoa and Vegetable Stir-Fry**:
   - 1 cup quinoa
   - 2 cups mixed vegetables (broccoli, bell pepper, carrots)
   - 2 tablespoons soy sauce
   - 1 tablespoon olive oil
   - 1 garlic clove, minced
   Cook quinoa as directed. Sauté vegetables and garlic in olive oil,

mix in quinoa and soy sauce, and stir well.

3. **Grilled Lemon Herb Chicken**:
   - 2 chicken breasts
   - Juice of 1 lemon
   - 1 teaspoon dried herbs (oregano or thyme)
   - Salt and pepper to taste
   Marinate chicken with lemon juice, herbs, salt, and pepper. Grill until fully cooked.

Resources for Further Exploration

- **Books**: Look for books focusing on nutrition, fitness, and mental wellness to deepen your understanding.

- **Websites**: Sites like Healthline, Mayo Clinic, and WebMD offer reliable health information and tips.

- **Apps**: Use fitness and meal-tracking apps to monitor your progress and stay committed.

With these recipes and resources, you're equipped to continue your journey towards a healthier you. Keep exploring, experimenting, and enjoying your path to wellness!

Author's Note

Dear Reader,

Thank you for embarking on this transformative journey with me through "Quick Fit: 21 Days to a Leaner You." This book was born out of my personal experiences and the lessons I've learned in striving for a healthier, more balanced life. My aim was not only to guide you through a short-term challenge but to equip you with the knowledge and habits necessary for sustained health and wellness.

The strategies outlined in this book are designed to be adaptable and flexible, recognizing that each person's journey is unique. I encourage you to customize these recommendations to fit your personal preferences, lifestyle, and goals. Remember, the key to success is consistency, not perfection. It's about making better choices more often, not about adhering flawlessly to a program. As you continue beyond these 21 days, remember that setbacks are part of the process. Embrace them as opportunities for learning and growth. Keep pushing forward, stay curious, and remain patient with yourself. Health is a lifelong journey.

Lastly, I am grateful for the opportunity to share this path with

you. May you find joy in every step of your ongoing adventure towards a healthier you.
Warm regards,
Spencer Whitelow
Here's a shopping list focused on healthy and nutritious snacks:
1. **Fresh Fruits**:
   - Apples
   - Bananas
   - Oranges
   - Berries (strawberries, blueberries, raspberries)
2. **Vegetables**:
   - Baby carrots
   - Celery sticks
   - Cherry tomatoes
   - Cucumbers
3. **Nuts and Seeds**:
   - Almonds
   - Walnuts
   - Sunflower seeds

  - Pumpkin seeds
4. **Protein Snacks**:
   - Greek yogurt
   - Cottage cheese
   - Hard-boiled eggs
   - Jerky (beef or turkey)
5. **Whole Grains**:
   - Whole grain crackers
   - Rice cakes
   - Popcorn (air-popped)
6. **Dips and Spreads**:
   - Hummus
   - Guacamole
   - Almond butter
   - Salsa
7. **Miscellaneous**:
   - Dark chocolate (at least 70% cocoa)
   - Dried fruit (no added sugar)
   - Roasted chickpeas
   - Seaweed snacks

These snacks are not only delicious but also provide a good mix of carbohydrates, protein, and healthy fats to keep you energized and satisfied between meals. Here's a comprehensive shopping list that covers your needs for vegetables, meats, and some staple items to ensure you have a well-rounded pantry and fridge:
Vegetables:
1. **Leafy Greens**:
   - Spinach
   - Kale
   - Romaine lettuce
2. **Cruciferous Vegetables**:
   - Broccoli
   - Cauliflower
   - Brussels sprouts
3. **Root Vegetables**:
   - Carrots
   - Beets

- Sweet potatoes
4. **Alliums**:
- Onions
- Garlic
- Leeks
5. **Versatile Veggies**:
- Bell peppers
- Zucchini
- Mushrooms
6. **Others**:
- Asparagus
- Cucumbers
- Tomatoes
Meats:
1. **Poultry**:
- Chicken breasts
- Chicken thighs
- Turkey
2. **Beef**:
- Ground beef
- Steak (e.g., sirloin, ribeye)
3. **Pork**:

    - Pork chops
    - Bacon
4. **Seafood**:
    - Salmon
    - Shrimp
    - Tilapia
5. **Other Proteins**:
    - Eggs
    - Tofu (for plant-based protein)
Staples:
1. **Grains**:
    - Rice (brown and white)
    - Quinoa
    - Pasta (whole grain or regular)
2. **Oils and Fats**:
    - Olive oil
    - Butter
    - Coconut oil
3. **Dairy**:
    - Milk
    - Cheese (various types)
    - Yogurt

4. **Canned and Jarred**:
   - Canned beans (black beans, chickpeas)
   - Canned tomatoes
   - Pickles
5. **Herbs and Spices**:
   - Salt and black pepper
   - Basil
   - Oregano
   - Cinnamon
6. **Condiments**:
   - Mustard
   - Ketchup
   - Soy sauce

This list should cover a variety of meals and recipes, providing both fresh ingredients and pantry essentials. Adjust quantities and specifics to match your dietary preferences and needs.

Here's a one-week meal plan that includes a variety of dishes to keep things interesting and nutritionally balanced. This plan assumes three main meals per day plus optional snacks.

Day 1:
- **Breakfast**: Greek yogurt with honey, almonds, and berries.
- **Lunch**: Grilled chicken salad with mixed greens, cherry tomatoes, avocado, and vinaigrette.
- **Dinner**: Baked salmon with garlic lemon butter sauce, steamed broccoli, and quinoa.
- **Snack**: Carrot sticks and hummus.

Day 2:
- **Breakfast**: Oatmeal topped with sliced bananas and a sprinkle of cinnamon.
- **Lunch**: Turkey and cheese sandwich on whole grain bread

with lettuce and tomato; side of cucumber slices.
- **Dinner**: Stir-fried beef with bell peppers and onions over brown rice.
- **Snack**: An apple and a handful of walnuts.
Day 3:
- **Breakfast**: Smoothie with spinach, protein powder, a banana, and almond milk.
- **Lunch**: Quinoa salad with chickpeas, cucumber, tomato, feta cheese, and a lemon-tahini dressing.
- **Dinner**: Pork chops with sweet potato mash and sautéed green beans.
- **Snack**: Greek yogurt with a dash of vanilla and fresh berries.
Day 4:

- **Breakfast**: Scrambled eggs with spinach and mushrooms; whole-grain toast.
- **Lunch**: Baked tilapia with a side salad and vinaigrette.
- **Dinner**: Pasta with marinara sauce, ground turkey, and a side of roasted asparagus.
- **Snack**: A peach and a small handful of almonds.
Day 5:
- **Breakfast**: Cottage cheese with sliced peaches and a drizzle of honey.
- **Lunch**: Chicken wrap with whole grain tortilla, lettuce, shredded carrots, and Caesar dressing.
- **Dinner**: Shrimp and vegetable stir-fry with a side of jasmine rice.
- **Snack**: Bell pepper strips and guacamole.

Day 6:
- **Breakfast**: Blueberry pancakes made with whole grain flour, topped with real maple syrup.
- **Lunch**: Lentil soup with a side of whole-grain crackers.
- **Dinner**: Grilled steak with baked potatoes and a side of steamed cauliflower.
- **Snack**: An orange and a few squares of dark chocolate.
Day 7:
- **Breakfast**: Bagel with cream cheese and smoked salmon; capers and onions optional.
- **Lunch**: Greek salad with mixed greens, olives, cucumber, tomato, and grilled chicken.
- **Dinner**: Homemade pizza with a whole grain base, topped with mozzarella, tomatoes, and basil.

- **Snack**: Mixed nuts and dried fruit.

Feel free to adjust the meals based on your dietary preferences, allergies, or specific nutritional needs. This meal plan is designed to provide a balanced mix of proteins, carbohydrates, and fats along with a good amount of fruits and vegetables to ensure a range of nutrients.